COMPLETE GUIDE TO DENTAL BRIDGE PLACEMENT

Comprehensive Manual To Restoring Smiles, Improving Oral Health, And Ensuring Long Lasting Tooth Solutions

DR. BRUNO HORAN

Copyright © 2023 by Dr. Bruno Horan

All rights reserved. Except for brief quotations embodied in critical reviews and certain other noncommercial uses permitted by copyright law, no part of this publication may be reproduced, distributed, or transmitted in any form or by any means, Including photocopying, recording, or other electronic or mechanical methods, without the prior written permission of the publisher.

Disclaimer:

The information provided in this book, is intended for general informational purposes only and should not be considered as professional advice.

The author has made every effort to ensure the accuracy of the information presented. However, readers are advised to consult with a qualified healthcare professional before attempting any herbal remedies or making significant changes to their wellness routine. Individual health conditions vary, and what may be suitable for one person may not be appropriate for another.

It is important to note that the author is not in any endorsement deal, partnership, or affiliation with any organization, brand, or company mentioned in this book. Any references to specific products or services are based on the author's personal experience or general knowledge and do not imply an endorsement or promotion of those products or services

Contents

CHAPTER ONE 19
EVALUATING AND DIAGNOSING 19
First Consultation Processes 19
Dental Examinations And Imaging Methods 20
Assessing Patient Appropriateness 21
Dental Bridge Diagnostic Standards 21
Personalization And Scheduling Of Treatment 22

CHAPTER TWO 25
READYING TO INSTAL A DENTAL BRIDGE 25
Teeth Cleaning Procedures 25
Pre-Operative Guidelines 26
Dietary Suggestions 27
Techniques For Pain Management 28
Psychological Readiness For The Operation 30

CHAPTER THREE 33
STEPS IN THE PROCEDURE 33
Options For Anesthesia And Sedation 33
Making Impressions And Preparing Teeth 35
Temporary Bridge Installation 37

CHAPTER FOUR 39
AFTER PROCEDURE CARE 39
Quick Post-Procedure Treatment 39

Medications And Pain Management 40

Dental Hygiene Procedures 41

Rescheduled Appointments 42

CHAPTER FIVE 45
PERMANENT MAINTENANCE 45
Daily Practices For Oral Hygiene 45

Expert Dental Cleanings 46

Nutritional Aspects 47

Early Identification And Resolution Of Problems . 48

Bridge Durability And Releasing 49

CHAPTER SIX 51
MANAGING DIFFICULTIES 51
Typical Issues And Their Root Causes 51

Handling Pain And Discomfiture 52

Controlling Infections And Ruptures 53

Fixing And Replacing Bridge Damage 54

When To Get Expert Assistance 55

CHAPTER SEVEN ... 57
CASE STUDIES AND PATIENT STORIES ... 57
Actual Patient Experiences ... 57
Common Problems And Their Fixes ... 58
Achievements ... 60
Knowledge Acquired ... 61
CHAPTER EIGHT ... 65
QUESTIONS ASKED REGULARLY ... 65
How Long Does A Dental Bridge Last? ... 65
How Should A Dental Bridge Be Maintained? ... 66
Can Someone Wearing A Dental Bridge Eat Normally? ... 67
When Using A Dental Bridge, Are There Any Food Restrictions? ... 70

CONCERNING THIS BOOK

"Dental Bridge Placement" provides a thorough examination of dental bridge operations from conception to long-term maintenance, making it a vital resource for both patients and dental professionals. The first section of the book provides a comprehensive overview of dental bridges, outlining their historical evolution as well as the different kinds and materials that are employed in contemporary dentistry. This basic information is essential because it lays the groundwork for understanding the many advantages of dental bridges, as well as the particular applications and situations in which they should not be used.

The assessment and diagnosis part outlines the methods for initial consultations, dental exams, and imaging techniques. It also dives into the crucial beginning steps of dental bridge placement. This section highlights how crucial it is to determine diagnostic criteria and assess patient eligibility to guarantee that every patient receives a customized treatment plan that caters to their particular requirements. Careful preparation is essential to the effective customization and implementation of the treatment.

The process is carefully explained, including the necessary pre-operative measures such as food advice, pain management techniques, and dental hygiene practices. This part also discusses the psychological preparation that patients must undergo to give them a comprehensive grasp of what to expect. This helps patients feel less anxious and cooperate better during the process.

The comprehensive, step-by-step guide provides vital insights into the process of placing both temporary and permanent bridges, as well as information on anesthesia and sedative choices, dental preparation, and taking impressions. This section helps to build confidence and transparency by ensuring that dental professionals can perform the procedure precisely and by providing patients with a deeper understanding of the technical aspects involved.

The book provides thorough instructions for immediate post-procedure care, pain management, and continuing oral hygiene habits. Post-procedure care is essential to the successful placement of dental bridges. It emphasizes the value of follow-up visits and informs patients about possible problems' warning signs, enabling proactive management and timely intervention when needed.

Comprehensive information about the long-term upkeep of dental bridges is included, along with helpful suggestions for regular dental cleanings, professional oral hygiene, and dietary adjustments. The book offers ways for managing replacements and maintaining bridge longevity, both of which are critical for extending the lifespan of the structure.

The care of complications is also included in the text, along with solutions for typical problems like pain, infections, and bridge damage. Patients are better able to take care of their oral health and keep their dental bridges in top shape when they are given guidance on when to seek professional assistance.

The book's patient stories and case studies, which provide real-life experiences, difficulties encountered, and solutions discovered, enhance its technical content. These personal accounts offer a motivating and relevant perspective, demonstrating the life-changing power of dental bridges.

Common patient concerns are addressed in a section dedicated to frequently asked questions, with succinct, understandable responses that promote well-informed decision-making. To give patients the knowledge they need to confidently maintain their oral health, this part addresses practical topics such as the lifespan of a dental bridge, care procedures, dietary limitations, and troubleshooting advice.

Overview of Dental Bridges

Synopsis and Background

Since ancient times, dental bridges have been used to replace lost teeth and improve the appearance and functionality of the mouth. Early dental bridges were made of materials like gold and ivory in ancient civilizations when the idea of restoring lost teeth first emerged. On the other hand, as dental technology has advanced, modern dental bridges have changed dramatically, providing patients with more practical, long-lasting, and aesthetically acceptable solutions. Modern dental bridges are expertly made to ensure a secure fit and a natural look, improving people's confidence and general oral health.

Dental Bridge Types and Material Selection

Dental bridges come in a variety of forms, each intended to address a particular set of circumstances and demands. The most typical kinds consist of:

Conventional Bridges: The most common kind, these includes creating a pontic (fake tooth) in between the crowns for the teeth on each side of the missing tooth. They usually have a natural appearance and great durability because they are comprised of materials like porcelain fused to metal or ceramics.

When there are neighboring teeth on just one side of the lost tooth or teeth, cantilever bridges are utilized. These are less prevalent and are typically utilized on less stressed parts of the mouth, including the front teeth.

Maryland Bonded Bridges: Often referred to as resin-bonded bridges, these are composed of gums and plastic teeth that are held up by a porcelain or metal framework. The bridge's porcelain or metal wings are cemented to your natural teeth on either side.

Bridges supported by implants are utilized in cases where multiple teeth are lost. These bridges are supported by dental implants rather than crowns or frames.

Dental bridges can be made of gold, alloys, porcelain, or a combination of these materials; the selection of these materials is contingent upon several factors, including the replacement tooth's function, the location of the missing tooth, and cosmetic preferences.

Dental Bridges' Advantages

For those who lack teeth, dental bridges can greatly enhance their quality of life with their many advantages. Among the main advantages are:

Restored Functionality: Missing teeth can make it difficult to chew and speak normally. Bridges help to restore these abilities.

Aesthetic Improvement: Your smile and general face appearance are improved by their natural-looking solution that melds in perfectly with the rest of your teeth.

Preserving Dental Structure:

Bridges preserve your facial structure and keep your remaining teeth from moving out of place by filling the space left by a lost tooth.

Long-Lasting Solution: Dental bridges are a dependable and long-lasting replacement for lost teeth that, with care, can survive for many years.

Better Oral Health: Bridges can help lower the risk of gum disease and tooth decay in neighboring teeth by substituting missing teeth.

Contraindications and Indications

Patients with one or more missing teeth and usually good oral health are candidates for dental bridges. Particular signs consist of:

Single or Multiple Missing Teeth: If the surrounding teeth are robust and in good condition, this option is best for patients who are missing one or more teeth.

Healthy Adjacent Teeth: For the bridge to be supported, the teeth next to the missing tooth must be in sufficient condition.

Good General Oral Health: For the bridge to be supported, patients need to maintain good gum health and oral cleanliness.

Dental bridge contraindications include the following:

Severe Gum Disease: Until the issue is treated, patients with active periodontal disease might not be suitable candidates.

Inadequate Bone Support: Before considering a bridge, patients with inadequate bone to support the bridge may need to undergo additional therapies, such as bone grafting.

Adjacent teeth that are decaying or damaged: Adjacent teeth that are weak or decayed may not be able to support a bridge.

Remnants of Dental Bridges

Depending on their unique requirements and circumstances, individuals may want to explore one of the many alternatives to dental bridges. Among them are:

Dental implants: A common substitute, implants offer a long-term fix that resembles the root of a real tooth. They can maintain jawbone density and do not require support from neighboring teeth.

Partial Dentures: Patients who would like to have a non-permanent solution can consider removable partial dentures. They might not provide the same stability as bridges or implants, but they are simple to remove and clean.

Resin-Bonded Bridges: These are a fantastic alternative for missing front teeth because they require less surgery than regular bridges. They employ a metal framework that is cemented to the teeth next to it.

Absence of Treatment: Although it can result in further dental problems like shifted teeth and biting disorders, people occasionally decide not to have a lost tooth replaced.

The position of the missing tooth, the patient's oral health, budget, and personal preferences are just a few of the variables that influence the decision. Each option has pros and downsides of its own.

CHAPTER ONE

EVALUATING AND DIAGNOSING

First Consultation Processes

The dentist will first go through your medical history and dental issues during the initial appointment for the implantation of a dental bridge.

This is an important stage since it clarifies any current conditions that could impact the course of treatment. You'll be able to talk about your expectations for the dental bridge and ask any questions you may have.

To evaluate the general condition of your oral cavity, the dentist will perform a comprehensive examination of your teeth and gums.

During this inspection, it can be necessary to look for cavities, and gum disease, and assess the health of the neighboring teeth that will support the bridge.

The quantity and quality of bone structure in the region where the bridge will be positioned will also be assessed by the dentist.

Dental Examinations And Imaging Methods

A variety of imaging techniques may be used to precisely plan where your dental bridge will be placed. X-rays give the dentist precise pictures of the teeth and the underlying bone structure, which they can use to find any hidden problems that could affect how well the bridge works.

A CT scan may be suggested in specific circumstances to provide a three-dimensional image of the region.

Furthermore, dental putty or digital scanning equipment will be used to take impressions of your teeth.

To fabricate a dental bridge that fits you perfectly, an exact model of your mouth must be created using these impressions.

These models will be used by the dentist to create a bridge that is identical to your real teeth in terms of size, shape, and color.

Assessing Patient Appropriateness

Dental bridges are not appropriate for every patient. The state of neighboring teeth, bone structure, and general oral health are all important considerations when assessing appropriateness.

The dentist will determine whether your gums and remaining teeth are in good enough condition to sustain a bridge during the examination.

Before putting in a bridge, patients with severe gum disease or low bone mass could need further therapies.

Dental Bridge Diagnostic Standards

To guarantee that a dental bridge will both function well and appear natural, diagnostic criteria for dental bridges entail a thorough examination of multiple variables.

The dentist will evaluate the stability of nearby teeth, the location of missing teeth, and the quantity and condition of missing teeth that require replacement. To make sure that the bridge won't obstruct your normal ability to chew, the dentist will also take into account the alignment of your bite and jaw movement.

Personalization And Scheduling Of Treatment

Following the completion of all diagnostic evaluations, the dentist will create a customized treatment plan based on your unique requirements.

The procedures for setting up and preparing the dental bridge will be described in this design. The process of customizing a bridge includes choosing the right materials (metal, porcelain, or ceramic) to best resemble your original teeth.

The dentist will go over the procedure's schedule, any possible risks or issues, and post-treatment care recommendations during the treatment planning step. We'll consider your preferences and feedback to make sure the finished product lives up to your expectations.

The aim is to design a dental bridge that smoothly improves the appearance of your smile while simultaneously restoring function.

CHAPTER TWO

READYING TO INSTAL A DENTAL BRIDGE

Teeth Cleaning Procedures

It is essential to practice good oral hygiene to get ready for the insertion of a dental bridge. Using fluoride toothpaste and brushing your teeth thoroughly twice a day will help get rid of plaque and germs that can lead to decay and gum disease. All of the surfaces of your teeth, particularly the regions along the gum line and the bridge, should be gently cleaned with a toothbrush with soft bristles. Flossing is similarly vital since, once the bridge is inserted, it gets rid of food particles and plaque from under the bridge.

Use an antibacterial mouthwash that your dentist has prescribed in addition to brushing and flossing. This can assist in maintaining the health of your gums and further minimize oral bacteria. Make sure to give special attention to and thoroughly clean any locations where the bridge will be installed.

In addition, your dentist might advise getting a professional cleaning during this preparatory period. This guarantees that before the bridge insertion process, your teeth and gums are in the best possible state. Following bridge placement, you can lessen the chance of issues and aid in the healing process by adhering to a regular dental cleaning regimen.

Pre-Operative Guidelines

Your dentist will provide you with clear preparation instructions before your dental bridge placement operation. These guidelines might specify if you need to fast before the surgery, especially if you'll be under anesthesia or sedation. It is usually the case that you will be instructed to fast for a predetermined amount of time before your visit.

You must adhere strictly to these directions to maximize safety and guarantee the success of your surgery. If you take any drugs, especially blood thinners, your dentist could advise modifying them to lower your risk of bleeding during and after the treatment. Make sure your dentist knows about all the medications you take at the moment.

Antibiotics may occasionally be prescribed by your dentist as a preventive precaution, particularly if you have a history of certain medical disorders or if infection is a worry. Complication risk is decreased when these drugs are used as prescribed.

Dietary Suggestions

It's critical to pay attention to your food after getting a dental bridge placed to support healing and preserve the new bridge. You might have to limit your diet to soft meals that don't need much chewing right after the treatment. Yogurt, mashed potatoes, smoothies, and soup are a few examples.

Steer clear of foods that are hard, sticky, or crunchy since they may damage or dislodge the bridge. As your dentist instructs, you can progressively add firmer foods back into your diet over time. During the first healing phase, you can further safeguard the bridge by chewing on the side of your mouth opposite the one where it was inserted.

Drinking lots of water to stay hydrated also promotes general oral health and can speed up the healing process.

See your dentist for individualized suggestions based on your unique needs if you have any specific dietary inquiries or concerns.

Techniques For Pain Management

It's critical to control pain and discomfort following dental bridge implantation to promote general comfort and healing. To aid with any discomfort or sensitivity, your dentist could suggest over-the-counter medications such as acetaminophen or ibuprofen.

For more severe suffering, your dentist may occasionally recommend stronger painkillers. Alcohol consumption while taking these medications might raise the chance of side effects and interfere with their effectiveness, so it's vital to follow the directions properly.

Numbness and swelling can also be lessened by placing an ice pack close to the treatment region on the outside of your face. As needed, apply the ice pack multiple times a day for 15 to 20 minutes at a time.

As was previously said, practicing proper dental hygiene can also help to lessen the discomfort by averting any possible side effects including gum inflammation or infection.

Psychological Readiness For The Operation

Anxiety can be reduced and a more seamless procedure can be achieved by feeling psychologically and emotionally ready for dental bridge implantation. Before any dental operation, it's normal to feel anxious, but being prepared can help reduce your anxiety.

Talk to your dentist in advance about any worries or fears you may have. They can address any queries you might have, clarify the stages needed, and offer information on the process. Anxiety can be decreased by being aware of the process and setting reasonable expectations.

Before and during the treatment, practice relaxation techniques like deep breathing or listening to soothing music.

To assist patients to unwind and divert themselves during treatment, several dental clinics additionally provide amenities like TVs or headphones.

Imagine a successful outcome and concentrate on the advantages of receiving a dental bridge. Remember that your dentist and their staff are accustomed to doing this operation and have plenty of experience making sure patients are comfortable and safe.

You may assist in guaranteeing a successful dental bridge placement treatment and a pain-free recovery process by mentally preparing yourself and adhering to the prescribed oral hygiene routines, dietary requirements, and pre-surgical instructions.

CHAPTER THREE

STEPS IN THE PROCEDURE

Options For Anesthesia And Sedation

To ensure a comfortable dental bridge placement process, anesthesia and sedation are essential. Your dentist will go over the many alternatives available to control discomfort and anxiety during the treatment with you before starting. These choices include sedative treatments that can help you relax or even fall asleep during the surgery, as well as local anesthesia, which numbs only the region being worked on.

Usually, an injection is used to provide local anesthetic close to the dental procedure site. It ensures that you experience little to no discomfort during the teeth preparation and impression-taking stages by blocking the nerves that perceive or transmit pain. Before the injection, your dentist could apply a topical numbing gel to reduce your level of discomfort.

Sedation solutions could be suggested for patients who need substantial dental procedures or who suffer from severe anxiety.

These can be intravenous (IV) sedation given straight into the circulation to produce deeper relaxation, or oral sedatives taken before to the consultation to induce a relaxed condition. Your dentist will evaluate your anxiety levels and medical history to decide the best sedation option for you.

Your vital signs and comfort will be continuously monitored by skilled dental professionals throughout the process.

This guarantees that the sedation or anesthetic is safe and effective for the duration of the dental bridge installation procedure. If sedation was used during the procedure, you will be watched until you are completely conscious and prepared to return home.

Making Impressions And Preparing Teeth

To ensure a proper fit and the lifetime of your new dental bridge, preparing your teeth and taking an impression are essential phases in the dental bridge placement process.

The abutment teeth, which will support the dental bridge, must first be carefully shaped. This is taking out a tiny bit of enamel to make room for the bridge and make sure it fits snugly.

After that, molds, or impressions, are made of the prepared teeth. The precise alignment and form of the abutment teeth, together with the surrounding gum tissue, are captured in these impressions.

Since these impressions are used as a guide to create your unique dental bridge, accuracy is essential. Digital scanning is one of the modern methods that can be used to make extremely accurate 3D photos of your teeth without the mess of traditional impression materials.

After being taken, the impressions are shipped to a dental laboratory where they are used by qualified experts to create both your permanent and temporary dental bridges.

While the ultimate bridge is being painstakingly made to guarantee ideal appearance and functioning, the temporary bridge is designed to shield the exposed teeth and gums.

Your dentist will make sure you are at ease and aware of every step of the tooth preparation and impression-taking procedure.

To guarantee a seamless transition to the following stage, any worries regarding tooth discomfort, the fit of the dental bridge, or the entire treatment can be swiftly addressed.

Temporary Bridge Installation

To provide protection and aesthetics while the final bridge is being built, temporary bridge installation is an essential interim stage in dental bridge treatment. Your dentist will carefully fit and cement a temporary bridge onto the prepared abutment teeth right after preparing the teeth and obtaining an imprint of the teeth.

The temporary bridge fulfills several crucial functions. It shields the exposed teeth and gums from potential harm and sensitivity while you wait for the last bridge to be completed.

During this transitional phase, it also helps keep the neighboring teeth in alignment and maintains normal chewing and biting functions.

The temporary bridge is made to be easily removed once the permanent bridge is completed, even though it is sturdy enough for regular daily use.

To ensure the lifetime of your temporary bridge and your comfort, your dentist will provide you with detailed instructions on how to take care of it, including dietary restrictions and dental hygiene guidelines.

Your dentist may arrange a follow-up visit during the temporary bridge phase to check on your recovery and make sure the temporary bridge is operating as intended. During this appointment, the temporary bridge can also have any necessary modifications performed to improve fit and comfort.

CHAPTER FOUR

AFTER PROCEDURE CARE

Quick Post-Procedure Treatment

It is imperative to adhere to specific maintenance guidelines following dental bridge implantation to promote good healing and bridge lifetime.

You can be given gauze by your dentist to stop any small bleeding that might happen at the implantation site. Some soreness or swelling in the vicinity of the bridge's placement is typical. Any soreness and swelling can be lessened by externally applying an ice pack.

After the procedure, refrain from eating on the side of your mouth where the bridge was placed. By taking this precaution, you can avoid putting undue pressure on the bridge and give the adhesive or cement time to fully cure.

To prevent sensitivity, your dentist might advise avoiding hot or cold foods and beverages at first.

Medications And Pain Management

After a dental bridge is placed, discomfort is usually controlled with over-the-counter medications such as acetaminophen or ibuprofen.

If more pain than you anticipated occurs, your dentist may recommend stronger painkillers. For successful pain management, it's critical to take prescription drugs exactly as your dentist prescribes.

Get in touch with your dentist right away if you suffer swelling that gets worse over time or if you feel extreme discomfort that does not go away with taking the recommended medication. These can indicate a problem that requires medical attention right now.

Dental Hygiene Procedures

For your dental bridge to last a long time, you must practice good oral hygiene. You can follow your dentist's instructions to properly clean the area surrounding the bridge.

Usually, this entails giving the bridge and neighboring teeth a gentle brushing with a toothbrush with soft bristles.

If regular brushing and flossing are unable to reach underneath the bridge, it may be recommended to use specialized floss threaders or interdental brushes.

It's crucial to keep up your regular flossing and twice-day brushing routines, giving close attention to the regions surrounding the bridge.

Maintaining good dental hygiene helps to avoid plaque accumulation, which over time can cause gum disease and weaken the integrity of the bridge.

Rescheduled Appointments

To track the healing process and make sure the bridge is operating properly, your dentist will arrange follow-up appointments. Your dentist may examine the bridge's fit, your bite, and the condition of the surrounding teeth and gums during these visits. Periodically, X-rays may be obtained to assess the bone structure beneath the bridge.

Additionally, follow-up appointments provide you the chance to discuss any worries or discomfort you may be experiencing and, if needed, make any necessary adjustments. For your dental bridge to be healthy and long-lasting, you must attend these checkups on time.

Signs of Difficulties to Be Aware of

Even if issues following the placement of a dental bridge are uncommon, it's crucial to recognize any warning signals. If you have severe pain that is not relieved by medicine, ongoing bleeding, swelling that gets worse over time, or if the bridge seems loose or unpleasant, get in touch with your dentist.

Additional warning signals to be aware of include persistently sensitive to hot or cold temperatures, bad taste or odor near the bridge, or infection-related symptoms like fever or enlarged lymph nodes. Early discovery of problems enables timely treatment, which can save more problems from arising and protect the integrity of your dental bridge.

CHAPTER FIVE

PERMANENT MAINTENANCE

Daily Practices For Oral Hygiene

For your dental bridge to last a long time, you must practice good oral hygiene. Including daily activities helps to maintain your bridge free of plaque accumulation, which can cause gum disease and other issues. It's crucial to brush your teeth using fluoride toothpaste and a soft-bristled toothbrush at least twice a day. Be sure to clean the area surrounding the abutment teeth that support the bridge as well as the gum line where the bridge joins your natural teeth.

Using floss or interdental brushes is essential for cleaning in between teeth and under bridges in addition to brushing. When flossing properly, the floss should be softly moved beneath the false tooth of the bridge as well as up and down the sides of each abutment tooth. This assists in removing food particles and plaque that may be missed by brushing alone. Including an antimicrobial mouthwash in your daily regimen can also aid in the reduction of bacteria and plaque, improving your dental health in general.

Expert Dental Cleanings

To keep your dental bridge in good condition, you must schedule routine cleaning appointments with your dentist. Your dentist or dental hygienist will clean the bridge and surrounding teeth carefully during these appointments, removing any plaque or tartar buildup that is difficult to remove at home. Additionally, by having your bridge professionally cleaned, your dentist can evaluate its integrity and spot any wear indicators or potential problems early on.

Your dentist may advise getting professional cleanings every six months, or more regularly if you have a history of tooth problems or certain disorders like gum disease. This will depend on your oral health needs. These check-ups add to the lifetime of your general dental health as well as maintaining the greatest possible appearance for your bridge.

Nutritional Aspects

Eating a balanced diet is crucial for the health of your dental bridge as well as for your general well-being. Preventing deterioration surrounding the bridge and safeguarding the integrity of the dental materials can be achieved by limiting the intake of sweet and acidic meals and beverages. Additionally, foods that are sticky or hard should be eaten carefully to prevent breaking or injuring the bridge.

Eating a diet high in vital minerals, such as calcium, vitamin D, and vitamin C, will maintain healthy teeth and gums, which will extend the life of your bridge. By rinsing away food particles and bacteria throughout the day, drinking lots of water helps maintain a healthy mouth environment. For particular advice regarding items that can impact your dental bridge, speak with your dentist if you have any dietary queries or concerns.

Early Identification And Resolution Of Problems

Taking early action to resolve any problems with your dental bridge is part of being proactive about your oral health. Sensitivity at the bridge, pain when chewing, or adjustments to the bridge's fit are typical indicators of possible issues. Make sure you get in quick to see your dentist if you have any of these symptoms or see anything out of the ordinary.

Early attention can stop little problems from growing into bigger ones that might need major repair or bridge replacement. To restore the functionality and aesthetics of your dental bridge, your dentist will do a comprehensive examination to identify the problem and make appropriate treatment recommendations.

Bridge Durability And Releasing

Your diet, routine dental care, and oral hygiene practices all affect how long your dental bridge will last. A well-made dental bridge can endure up to 15 years or longer with the right upkeep and care. To guarantee continuous functionality and beauty, the bridge may eventually need to be repaired or replaced due to normal wear and tear.

Your dentist can monitor the condition of your bridge and determine whether it needs to be adjusted or replaced with routine dental check-ups. Unexpected bridge replacement may be required due to several factors such as alterations in your bite alignment, deterioration of the bridge materials, or changes in your dental health. To preserve the durability of your dental bridge and your oral health, you and your dentist will collaborate closely to decide on the best course of action.

CHAPTER SIX

MANAGING DIFFICULTIES

Typical Issues And Their Root Causes

Although dental bridge placements are usually safe and successful, problems can occasionally arise, just like with any dental operation.

Sensitivity following the treatment is a common problem that usually results from the teeth and gums acclimating to the new bridge.

Patients may occasionally experience mild discomfort or irritation of the gums, particularly if there is a slight variation in the bite or if the bridge is not properly aligned.

The bridge's gradual weakening is another possible problem. This may occur if the bridge is under too much strain as a result of teeth grinding or biting on hard items, or if the cement used to secure the bridge does not adequately bind with the tooth enamel. Inadequate dental hygiene can also lead to issues like gum disease and decay surrounding the bridge, which may need more care to be resolved.

Handling Pain And Discomfiture

For a few days following dental bridge installation, some soreness or sensitivity is common. Usually, this soreness goes away as your mouth's tissues get used to the new bridge.

Ibuprofen and other over-the-counter painkillers can help with slight pain and discomfort during this time. Avoiding extremely hot or cold foods and beverages can also reduce sensitivity.

You must get in touch with your dentist if the discomfort continues or gets worse. They can inspect the bridge to make sure that the discomfort isn't being caused by problems with fit or alignment.

Occasionally, the issue might be resolved by making small changes to the bridge.

Controlling Infections And Ruptures

Although they are rare, infections and inflammations surrounding a dental bridge can happen, particularly if plaque and germs have accumulated beneath or around the bridge. Infection symptoms might include foul breath or an off taste in the mouth, as well as swelling, redness, or soreness in the gums surrounding the bridge.

It is essential to practice appropriate dental hygiene to control these problems. Plaque accumulation can be avoided by brushing and flossing the area surrounding the bridge twice a day. To lessen oral microorganisms, your dentist could also advise using an antimicrobial mouthwash.

If an infection does develop, your dentist might have to thoroughly clean the afflicted area and, if required, prescribe antibiotics. It is imperative to swiftly handle any indications of infection to avert additional consequences.

Fixing And Replacing Bridge Damage

A dental bridge may occasionally sustain damage from wear and tear over time, accidents, or decay beneath the bridge.

It's critical to contact your dentist right away if you discover any chips, cracks, or loose parts on your bridge. Ignoring damage can result in more issues down the road, like discomfort or tooth rot.

When repairing a damaged bridge, one must usually evaluate the amount of the damage and decide whether a straightforward repair will suffice or if a new bridge must be built.

Based on your unique circumstances, your dentist will assess the bridge's condition and suggest the best course of action.

When To Get Expert Assistance

Maintaining your oral health after receiving a dental bridge requires knowing when to seek professional assistance.

It's recommended to get in touch with your dentist if you have ongoing pain, irritation, or sensitivity that doesn't go away after a few days. They can assess the bridge and deal with any problems that might be contributing to your symptoms.

Likewise, you must seek immediate dental care if you observe any infection-related symptoms, such as swelling, redness, or unusual discharge surrounding the bridge. Prompt action can stop the infection from growing and developing more issues.

Additionally, make an appointment with your dentist right once if your bridge gets loose or damaged. Any problems with your dental bridge should be promptly addressed to maintain its durability and efficacy in repairing your smile.

You can make sure that your dental bridge lasts for many years and supports your general oral health by maintaining good oral hygiene and getting professional assistance when necessary.

CHAPTER SEVEN

CASE STUDIES AND PATIENT STORIES

Actual Patient Experiences

Patient narratives frequently offer priceless insights into the process of placing a dental bridge. A typical feeling that many patients have in common is their initial anxiety about the treatment. Many people are concerned about the pain or discomfort involved, but they find comfort in the skillful numbing treatments and gentle approach employed by skilled dental practitioners.

Emily, one of the patients, talked about how she had to get a dental bridge after a bad accident. Emily was first worried about the procedure, but she discovered that her dentist took the time to fully explain each step. Emily felt informed and supported from the first consultation to the final placement, which significantly reduced her worry. She emphasized the value of having an honest conversation with her dentist and expressed gratitude for the considerate way in which her issues were handled.

Despite his early misgivings, John, another patient, characterized his experience as constructive. Because of tooth deterioration, he required a dental bridge. John underlined how crucial it is to have faith in the dental team's knowledge. He discovered that his dentist gave solutions that suited his lifestyle and budget in addition to a clear strategy for the bridge's placement.

Common Problems And Their Fixes

Even with the development of dental technology, placing a dental bridge can present certain difficulties. During the preparation phase, when the teeth next to the gap are altered to make room for the bridge, patients frequently experience discomfort. Modern sedative methods and anesthetics, however, help to reduce any discomfort and provide a more comfortable procedure.

Maria, a patient who had a bridge placed, first had trouble with concerns about how her smile would look after the treatment.

To ensure a seamless fit, her dentist collaborated extensively with her to choose a bridge that matched the color and shape of her natural teeth. Maria felt more confident in her smile and her fears were allayed by this attention to detail.

The period of adjustment following bridge placement presents another potential challenge for patients. Some patients say they were first sensitive to the new structure or found it difficult to adjust.

Dentists frequently advise a limited time of adjustment so that any little discomfort can be swiftly resolved. Dentists can check the fit of the bridge and make any changes for optimal comfort and functionality by scheduling regular follow-up appointments.

Achievements

There are many success stories in the field of dental bridge implantation, demonstrating the life-changing effects on patients.

For example, Sarah was able to chew and speak normally again after getting a bridge to replace her lost teeth. She described how her quality of life and social confidence were greatly enhanced by the restored function.

The aesthetic advantages of Mark's dental bridge are the focal point of his success story. Being in a field where professionals interact with clients, Mark was self-conscious about the spaces between his teeth.

His dentist suggested a bridge that would blend in perfectly with his natural teeth, improving his appearance and restoring his confidence.

Knowledge Acquired

From patient experiences, the dental community and individuals thinking about placing a bridge can learn several important things.

The value of careful planning and consultation is one important lesson. Patients who are aware of the process and what to expect from it usually feel more assured and pleased with the outcome.

Furthermore, maintaining patient satisfaction is largely dependent on effective communication. Dentists who effectively customize treatment programs to each patient's needs are those who take the time to listen to their problems and preferences.

In addition to improving patient comfort, this individualized strategy also leads to improved long-term results.

Motivational Travels

Transformation and resiliency are frequently highlighted in inspirational dental bridge placement stories. Bridges are examples of cutting-edge dental treatments that gave patients like James, who had severe teeth issues because of their genetic makeup, newfound hope.

His transformation from unease and uncertainty to regained self-assurance is a source of inspiration for anyone dealing with comparable challenges.

Another motivational tale is that of Lisa, who used a bridge to restore her smile after overcoming her dread of dental work.

Her path included using patient-centered care and empathetic treatment to overcome her fear of the dentist. Lisa's metamorphosis demonstrated the transformative power of preventive dental health care.

Every patient's experience and case study about the placement of dental bridges illustrates distinct difficulties, customized solutions, and finally, the revolutionary potential of contemporary dentistry. These stories educate and motivate people who are thinking of getting dental bridges to improve their oral health and overall well-being.

CHAPTER EIGHT

QUESTIONS ASKED REGULARLY

How Long Does A Dental Bridge Last?

The type of dental bridge, oral hygiene habits, and general dental health are some of the variables that can affect how long a bridge lasts.

A well-maintained dental bridge can endure up to 15 years or more on average. The materials utilized, such as zirconia, all-ceramic, or porcelain fused to metal, each with unique characteristics and aesthetic attributes, affect the bridge's durability.

To keep an eye on the health of the bridge and the underlying teeth, routine dental examinations are essential.

Your dentist will examine the surrounding teeth and gums for any indications of wear, fit, or possible problems. By reducing gum disease and decay, regular dental care, such as brushing and flossing, can significantly increase the life of your dental bridge.

How Should A Dental Bridge Be Maintained?

For your dental bridge to be functional and long-lasting, proper maintenance is required. Here are some useful pointers to make sure your bridge stays in good shape:

Handle your dental bridge with the same care as you would a natural tooth. To clean the area around and beneath the bridge of plaque and food particles, use fluoride toothpaste and brush at least twice a day.

Using interdental brushes or dental floss threaders: These instruments facilitate the cleaning of difficult-to-reach spaces between teeth and beneath bridges.

Frequent dental visits: Make an appointment for routine cleanings and examinations to keep an eye on the condition of your bridge and the teeth around it.

Your dentist can identify any problems early and provide the required corrections or repairs.

Chewing on hard objects might cause damage to the bridge or cause it to come away. Steer clear of biting down on hard objects like ice, pencils, or nuts.

Keep up a healthy diet: Consuming a diet high in fruits and vegetables and balanced in calories promotes good dental health. Reducing the consumption of sugar-filled snacks and drinks can help prevent degradation near the edges of the bridge.

You can contribute to ensuring your dental bridge stays pleasant and functional for many years to come by adhering to these care recommendations and practicing proper oral hygiene.

Can Someone Wearing A Dental Bridge Eat Normally?

You can resume your normal eating routine after a period of adjustment to your dental bridge. It could take a little while for you to get used to how the bridge feels in your mouth at first. Once you are comfortable with the stability of your bridge, then you can reintroduce tougher or chewier meals, but start with softer foods first.

Like real teeth, dental bridges are made to endure typical biting and chewing forces. To avoid breaking or dislodging the bridge, you must, however, refrain from biting down on really hard materials or using your teeth as tools.

See your dentist right away for an assessment if you feel any pain or if the bridge feels loose when eating. To guarantee both your comfort and the bridge's lifetime, they can evaluate the fit and make any required alterations.

If I feel like my bridge is loose, what should I do?

It's critical to take immediate action to stop additional harm or discomfort if your dental bridge seems loose or moves when you bite or chew. These are actions that you can do:

Get in touch with your dentist: Make an appointment as soon as you can. To find the reason for the looseness, they will inspect the bridge and the teeth that support it.

Steer clear of chewing on that side: Steer clear of chewing on the side where the bridge feels loose to keep it from getting more unstable or damaged.

Uphold good oral hygiene by gently brushing and flossing the region surrounding the bridge. Keeping your mouth clean helps avoid more issues while you wait for your dentist visit.

A dental bridge's looseness may result from several things, including regular wear and tear over time, problems with the gums or supporting teeth, or unintentional injury. After evaluating the circumstances, your dentist will suggest the best course of action for securing or repairing the bridge to improve comfort and functionality.

When Using A Dental Bridge, Are There Any Food Restrictions?

Although the purpose of dental bridges is to replace lost chewing ability, there are some dietary guidelines to follow to extend their life and preserve your oral health:

Steer clear of excessively hard or sticky foods: Hard candies, ice cubes, and sticky foods like caramels should not be chewed on since they may break the bridge or cause it to come loose.

chop food into smaller pieces: To ease the strain on the bridge and neighboring teeth, chop tougher items, like apples or raw vegetables, into smaller, more manageable pieces.

Chew uniformly: To reduce stress on the bridge and provide balanced chewing forces, distribute food equally on both sides of your mouth.

Eat a range of nutrient-dense foods to improve general oral health by maintaining a balanced diet. Steer clear of sugar-filled snacks and drinks in excess as this can exacerbate the deterioration surrounding the bridge's edges.

You can help guarantee your dental bridge stays stable and functional for years to come by adhering to these dietary guidelines and maintaining proper oral hygiene. This will enable you to enjoy a wide variety of foods without discomfort or difficulties.